HELP YOURSELF

TO

POSITIVE MENTAL

HEALTH

Howard Rosenthal, Ed.D.
Joseph W. Hollis, Ed.D.

Accelerated Development, Inc.
A member of the Taylor & Francis Group

HELP YOURSELF TO POSITIVE MENTAL HEALTH

Technical Development: Cynthia Long
Marguerite Mader
Sheila Sheward

Library of Congress Cataloging-in-Publication Data

Rosenthal, Howard, 1952-
   Help yourself to positive mental health / Howard Rosenthal, Joseph
W.   Hollis.
      p.   cm.
      ISBN 1-55959-069-6
      1. Conduct of life. 2. Behavior modification. 3. Attitude change.
   4. Mental health. I. Hollis, Joseph William. II Title.
   BF637.C5R67 1994
   158' .1—dc20   94-19050
                                                                 CIP

LCN:94-19050
ISBN: 1-55959-069-6

Order additional copies from

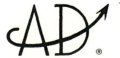

ACCELERATED DEVELOPMENT INC.
A member of the Taylor & Francis Group
325 Chestnut Street
Philadelphia, PA 19106

INTRODUCTION TO THE BOOK

Get ready for an exciting personal adventure that could change your life!

In this one-of-a-kind book, you'll discover 50 simple ideas teamed up with **specific activities** that you can use **immediately** to help yourself to positive mental health.

Here you'll discover **easy-to-understand techniques and specific suggestions** to combat depression, fear, loneliness, anger, poor self-image, undesirable habits, poor communication, relationship difficulties, and more. Step-by-step procedures are provided to help you implement ideas that will leave you feeling great!

But wait...we have even more good news for you. For years now, professional helping and even "pop psychology" has been plagued with jargon...large 25-cent words that you'd need a dictionary to spell and a speech teacher to pronounce for you.

For those of you who have taken an introductory psychology course, you already know what we're talking about. You've seen—and very likely been intimidated by—terms like id, ego, super ego, reciprocal inhibition, dissonance, sublimation, or countertransference.

Worse yet, the problem isn't solved even when you are familiar with the terminology, since many behavioral terms can have numerous meanings. It has been suggested, for example, that a current popular term, "codependency," could refer to some 254 separate characteristics!!! (Lots of luck figuring that one out.) Well, relax. You can place your dictionaries of psychology and psychiatry back on the bookshelf You won't be needing them to comprehend this book.

We've done everything in our power to keep the material "jargon-free." When we do mention a famous theorist or a technical term (such as "desensitization" or "dichotomous thinking"), we go on to explain it in plain everyday English.

Now because we firmly believe that what we have to say is extremely important, we don't want you to lose interest. Therefore, we intentionally have written this book in an exciting new "user-friendly," conversational style that makes the material so lively and entertaining you won't want to put it down! But don't take our word for it; read the book and make us prove it to you. We think you'll be pleasantly surprised.

Just think of it this way. Imagine that for one evening you've cornered a couple of professional helpers. These guys have been around a while and really know the ropes. Between them, these two fellows have counseled hundreds of individuals, lectured to over 100,000 people, taught courses at various colleges and universities, and written numerous articles and books. You'll wine' em (with nonalcoholic beverages, of course) and dine 'em so you can pick their brains about what you can do to live a happier, more productive life. You're not interested in a bunch of useless complicated theories for gosh sakes...

YOU WANT ANSWERS!   YOU WANT RESULTS!
YOU WANT BETTER RELATIONSHIPS!
YOU WANT STRATEGIES THAT YOU
CAN IMPLEMENT NOW!

YOU WANT WHAT'S IN THIS BOOK!

HOW TO USE THIS BOOK TO IMPROVE YOUR LIFE RIGHT NOW

In this book, you'll be given things you can do to improve your mental health—50 of them, to be exact. Don't let the simplicity of these ideas fool you; they can be extremely effective.

The format is really quite simple. On the right page, you'll discover the basic idea (such as Use Role Reversal to Take the Sting out of a Nasty Argument). Then as you read the left page, you'll find a concise explanation (never longer than one page) that explains the concept and how to implement it. Plenty of actual examples and specific actions to take are outlined.

* Use the book yourself and help yourself to positive mental health.

* Share the information and activities with a trusted friend.

* If you're a professional counselor, therapist, youth specialist, peer counselor, or other helper, assign this book as therapeutic homework for your clients.

* If you're a group facilitator or classroom teacher, discuss the ideas in group, and then try performing some of the recommended activities as a group exercise. Participants then can implement the ideas outside the group and share their experiences.

* If you're studying to be a helper, try the suggestions yourself, and then discuss with your professor or practicum instructor how you could use them with your clients.

There's a revolution going on in the field of health. For the first time, we're being asked to exercise, quit smoking, and eat broccoli to achieve positive health. Doctors are saying: "You can help take charge of your own health." We believe you should do likewise with your mental health.

You can think of this book as broccoli for your mind, though we have this uncanny suspicion you'll find it a lot tastier.

With a warm hand clasp,

Dr. Howard Rosenthal & Dr. Joseph Hollis

NOTE: Proper names, locations, and descriptions have been changed to protect the confidentiality of our clients.

HELP

YOURSELF

Fifty Things to Improve

Your Mental Health

To reward yourself for doing the right thing sounds incredibly simple, but it works wonders. Behavioral scientists call it "positive reinforcement," and it can be used to strengthen or increase any behavior. Although the U.S. Air Force never took him up on it, the great psychologist, B.F. Skinner, seriously suggested that he could use reinforcement to make pigeons—yes pigeons—fly guided missiles during World War II. What's more, he was convinced that if the reinforcer (a reward) was administered properly, the birds would never make a mistake!

Now if a bird brain can do that, imagine what you could accomplish!

For reinforcement to do its thing, however, you must give yourself the reward immediately after performing the desirable act. (That's where our *monthly* paychecks fall painfully short.)

If, for example, you reinforce or reward yourself for doing your homework by purchasing a new scarf, make certain you purchase the scarf as soon as possible after completing the homework.

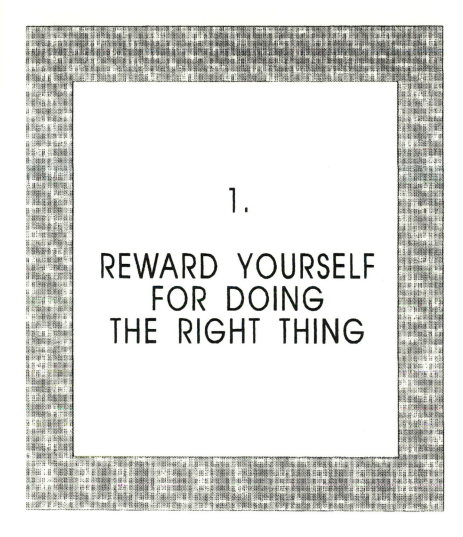

1.

REWARD YOURSELF
FOR DOING
THE RIGHT THING

"Got a problem?" ask the behavior modifiers. "Then why not rely on the Premack Principle by reinforcing a LPB with a HPB." If that sounds a little too complex, let us simplify it in plain everyday english.

Behavior modification expert David Premack discovered that one of the finest ways to strengthen or increase a low probability behavior (LPB) is by reinforcing or rewarding yourself with a high probability behavior (HPB). Aw, that still sounds too complicated; let's take a look at a typical situation.

Let's say that you have a report you need to finish. Let us further assume that this is a low probability behavior because you would rather do almost anything else before you'd work on that report. In other words, it's the last thing you really want to do.

According to the Premack Principle, your first step is to look for a behavior that you naturally enjoy, say drinking a chocolate milk shake with extra whip cream and a cherry. Anyway, in this example, gulping down the milk shake is a high probability behavior you can use to reinforce or reward yourself for working on your report.

You then would set up your own program in which you get to guzzle down your shake but only AFTER you finish say two or three pages of your report.

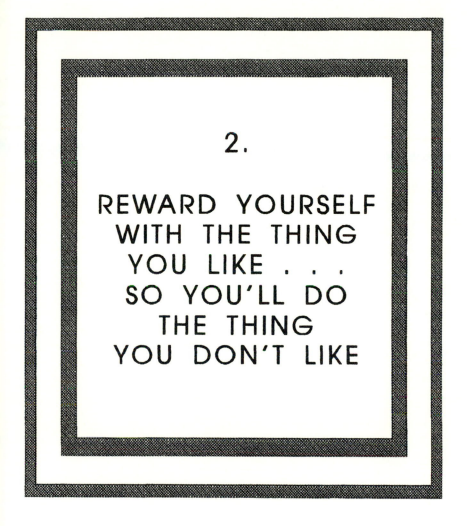

2.

REWARD YOURSELF
WITH THE THING
YOU LIKE . . .
SO YOU'LL DO
THE THING
YOU DON'T LIKE

From time to time, we all feel a little blue, sad, and down in the dumps. The next time it happens to you, why not prescribe a little exercise for yourself? A short walk, a little gardening, a low-impact dance class, or a spin on your exercise bike can be just what you need to boost your spirits.

It seems that regular moderate exercise increases a class of neurochemicals called catecholamines just like expensive antidepressant drugs do!

Yes, even evidence from space programs indicates that inactivity can cause depression while activity can help cure it.

But a word of warning: Just because a little bit is good doesn't mean a lot is better. Sports psychologist Dr. William Morgan, of the University of Wisconsin, discovered that extremely heavy exercise significantly increases depression. Thus, while a half-mile brisk walk could be beneficial, a 26-mile sprint could be emotional (not to mention physical) suicide!

So don't wait until you can spell the word "catecholamines" to begin (that could be a while, you know). Put on an old pair of tennis shoes and let's get a move on it.

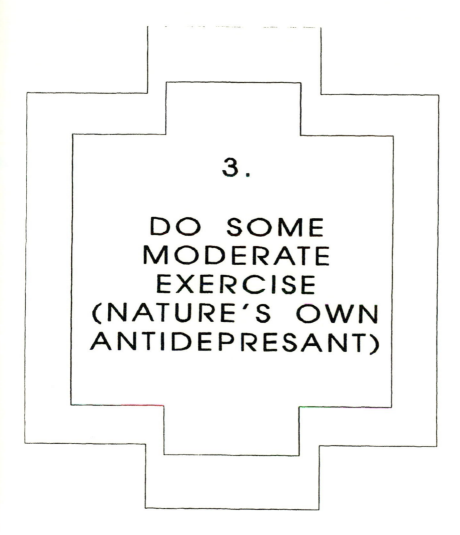

3.

DO SOME MODERATE EXERCISE (NATURE'S OWN ANTIDEPRESANT)

All over the country, treatment centers and practitioners have discovered the magic of journaling. Keeping a journal of your personal thoughts, feelings, ideas, and reactions allows you to step outside yourself so you can better evaluate your behavior and make the necessary changes. A situation that seemed impossible to cope with on Monday, often seems easy to tackle on Friday.

The mere act of putting your reactions in writing seems to be therapeutic for many individuals.

Moreover, many people discover that journaling enhances creativity.

And as if the aforementioned benefits weren't good enough, you'll be able to use your journal to monitor the progress you'll be making as you faithfully implement the wonderful ideas in this book.

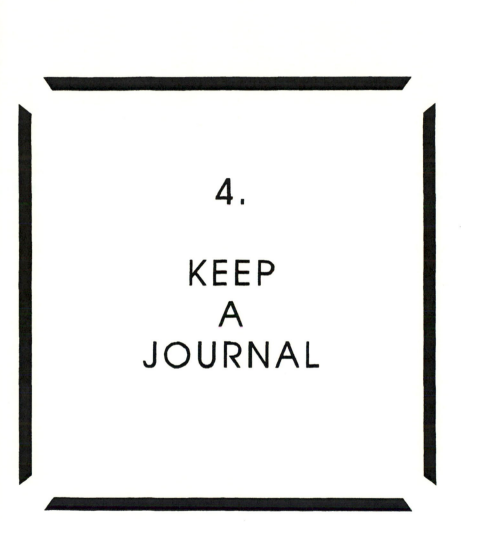

4.

KEEP
A
JOURNAL

Perhaps you'd like to ask your roommate's sister out on a date yet you don't have a clue how to begin. Maybe you believe you deserve a raise but you always seem a bit tongue-tied around your boss. And how can someone like you who never wants to hurt anybody's feelings tell your mother-in-law that she can't move into your spare bedroom?

Why not role-play the situation in advance with a friend? This will give you a chance to practice what you want to say in an emotionally safe environment. Your friend can give you feedback about how you really are coming across. Such feedback can help you fine-tune your approach.

Counselors call this valuable technique "behavior rehearsal," and it can be utilized in literally hundreds of practical situations.

Try it. This one's a winner even if you don't snare any academy awards.

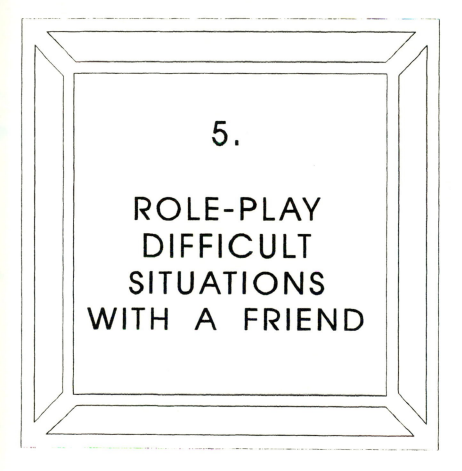

5.

ROLE-PLAY DIFFICULT SITUATIONS WITH A FRIEND

Here's a technique you can use to help yourself or someone you care about. It's called "behavioral contracting," or "self-contracting" when it applies to you exclusively. For some reason, the written word yields a tremendous amount of power. Just mention the word "contract" (perhaps because it has traditionally had legal connotations) and watch how quickly people's faces become serious.

Crisis centers throughout the nation have discovered that contracts actually exert enough clout to save a suicidal person. Some suicidal individuals have admitted forthrightly that the only reason they are still alive is that they decided to honor a behavioral contract that stated they would not harm themselves!

Many treatment centers for children, adolescents, and adults alike refuse to terminate a client until he or she (and sometimes the significant others) signs a contract. Many therapists including behavior therapists, reality therapists, and those practicing transactional analysis swear by the technique.

Contracts work best when (1) they are specific (e.g., I will not smoke more than two cigarettes during my eight-hour work shift), (2) they are teamed up with a reward (e.g., If I smoke two cigarettes or less during my eight-hour work shift, I will allow myself to see a movie of my choice), (3) all parties have input regarding the wording, (4) they are signed and dated by all parties involved, and (5) all parties involved are given a signed copy of the document.

Finally, put the contract in the most conspicuous place possible, say on the door of your refrigerator or the upper right hand side of your television screen!

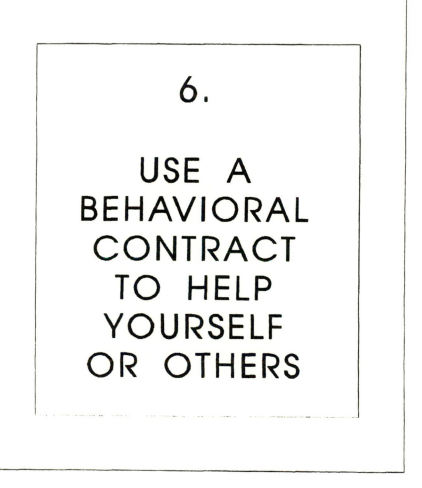

6.

USE A
BEHAVIORAL
CONTRACT
TO HELP
YOURSELF
OR OTHERS

After many years of research, the well-known psychologist Martin E.P. Seligman discovered that the difference between depressed people and happy people is not due merely to their life circumstances or what happens to them...it's based on their thinking. Simply put: Unhappy individuals are pessimistic, while those who feel good about themselves are optimistic.

Optimistic individuals are better able to overcome tragedy such as physical or sexual abuse. Optimistic patients with horrendous medical conditions like cancer or AIDS seem to live longer, and in some cases, their conditions subside. Optimistic athletes bounce back after a bad game. And amazing as it sounds, politicians who give optimistic political speeches tend to win more elections!

The exciting news is that counselors believe almost anyone can learn to be more optimistic. The trick is to work hard—really hard—in regard to changing those pessimistic thoughts and attitudes. Instead of thinking, "diets don't work," for example, you can change it to, "THIS diet doesn't work." The new revised optimistic thought, of course, implies that another diet might be exactly what you need.

Can this strategy really work? Two words provide the answer: Be optimistic!

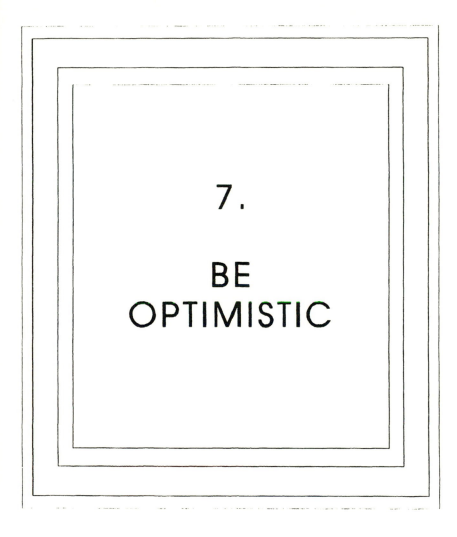

7.

BE
OPTIMISTIC

What did you say or think about yourself today? If it was anything like, "I'm stupid," "I'm fat," "I'm ugly," "I'm no good at math," "I never perform well in the clutch," "I'm not good with men," etc., etc., etc., then you're doing a hatchet job on yourself.

Negative labels lead to a poor self-image, and that's the last thing you want and/or need.

Think of some positive things about yourself. Stop cutting yourself down! If you define yourself in a negative manner, then you will very often behave "as if" the label is true!

Try living for an hour, a week, a month, or better still an entire year, without those old detrimental labels and see if your hidden potential doesn't begin to show its face.

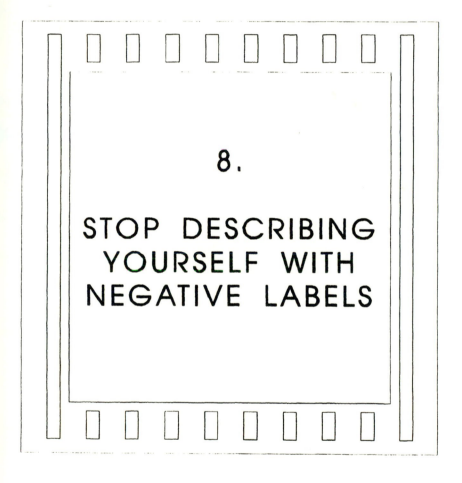

8.

STOP DESCRIBING
YOURSELF WITH
NEGATIVE LABELS

"I was born in the wrong era."

"My father never gave me the attention I needed."

"My third-hour economics professor is a jerk."

"My boss at work is a jerk!"

"Häagen-Dazs made me break my diet." (Oh, come now!)

"The devil made me do it."

Stop!!! Many mental health professionals insist that blame is a useless emotion. Why? Well the answer is easy.

Note that when you blame the year you were born, your father, your third hour professor, your boss, Häagen-Dazs, or the devil it's an excuse not to look at yourself. This translates to an excuse not to change your own behavior. Isn't that an interesting self-defeating dynamic!

Try tackling tough situations without blaming anybody or anything and watch life change for the better.

9.

STOP BLAMING OTHERS FOR YOUR DIFFICULTIES

A patient was hospitalized for anxiety and an inability to sleep. She emphasized that for the past six months she was so nervous she couldn't sleep a wink. She further informed the staff that she had been treated by numerous individuals and nothing ever had helped. With that, she challenged the staff by asking, "Well, what do you think you're going to do for me?"

She was told that her anxiety needed to be monitored, and she was instructed absolutely, positively, not to sleep, but rather to STAY UP ALL NIGHT AND HAVE THE BEST ANXIETY ATTACK POSSIBLE!

The next day the patient came to group therapy and announced that the technique failed: SHE HAD SLEPT LIKE A BABY!!!

Helping professionals call it "paradox," but your grandmother didn't believe in complicating the issue, so she merely referred to it as "reverse psychology."

Many parents who have fought with their teenagers to turn down the stereo have discovered that once they profess that they "like the music" and turn the stereo up even further so they can hear it better, their teen rebels and decides the volume is too loud! Please note that in this case, as well as the situation in the hospital, the individuals who implemented the reverse psychology got what they wanted.

So don't say you've tried everything until you give reverse psychology a whirl. One very serious word of caution, however, never use this technique in a situation where a person is threatening to hurt himself or someone else.

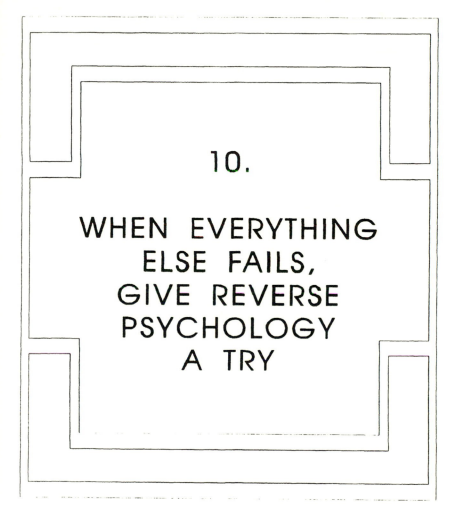

10.

WHEN EVERYTHING ELSE FAILS, GIVE REVERSE PSYCHOLOGY A TRY

Ponder the following questions. Has a friend ever said, "I'll call you for lunch" and then didn't follow through? Did someone you know ever remark, "Don't bother buying such and such, I'll give you mine"?

Now it's two years later and you're still waiting for your luncheon date and the amazing SUCH AND SUCH. Well, how do you feel about it? The answer can usually be summed up concisely in one word: disappointed! So how do others feel when you fail to follow through on your promises? Disappointed, of course!

Making and subsequently breaking promises is epidemic in this day and age. You should strive to break away from the disappointing "psychology of the average" when you're reaching for positive mental health.

You can begin by making a list of all the promises you've made to others. Then, one by one, begin to fulfill them (yes, even if it's been a while since you got somebody's hopes up).

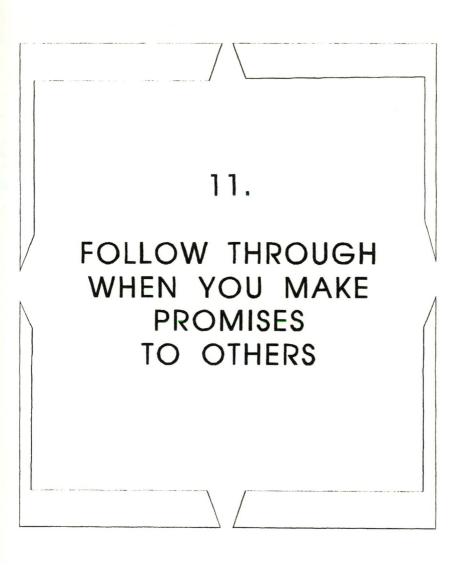

11.

FOLLOW THROUGH WHEN YOU MAKE PROMISES TO OTHERS

"I want to lose 57 pounds."

"I want to play pro ball."

"I'd like to attain three master's degrees."

All of the above are commendable goals. Unfortunately, after you've been striving for them for a short period of time, you may feel...well...overwhelmed. Simply put, they seem too big...too difficult..insurmountable...and ultimately just plain impossible!!!

When the word "impossible" reaches your brain, the likelihood is about 98% that you'll just give up on your dream.

Thus, instead of setting yourself up for failure, set yourself up for success by setting smaller goals that are realistic and easier to achieve. When you succeed at small goals it will give you confidence.

Vow to lose 2 pounds in the next 14 days. Go out for intramural football or see if you can make the 8th-grade team. Secure a course catalog or sign up for a single graduate course.

As you reach your small goals, you'll not only be moving toward your bigger goal, but you'll be developing a positive mind-set.

Yes, a journey of a thousand miles really does begin with the first step...and ideally a very small one at that.

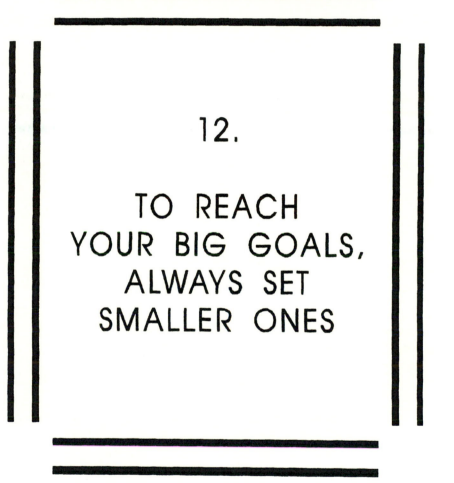

12.

TO REACH
YOUR BIG GOALS,
ALWAYS SET
SMALLER ONES

Mr. P was finally leaving the company after 23 years of service. As he cleaned out his desk, he threw out literally hundreds of useless papers, forms, and documents. None of them, as far as he was concerned, were worth the paper they were printed on. None of them, that is, except for two—two small memos where he had been complimented by his boss for jobs well done. These he would keep. These he would cherish forever.

Stop waiting! Stop assuming the person has heard it a million times! If you know somebody who deserves a compliment, give it to him or her!

This is the time to use a little Clint Eastwood psychology: Go ahead, make my day (while you make your own) with a compliment.

13.

GIVE
SOMEONE
A
COMPLIMENT

Now here's a dramatic self-help strategy! Act as if you are already the person you want to be.

If you are shy and don't like yourself, act as if you are outgoing. If you are sad and blue, act like you're happy and not depressed. Of course, you'll need to ask yourself: Precisely how would an outgoing individual or a happy person act?

A great psychologist named George Kelly once built a therapeutic school of helping known as "fixed role therapy" based on this technique. Begin by writing a page or two depicting how you'd like to be, and then act as if you already are that way.* Remember to read the sketch several times daily.

Try it out initially for just a few minutes, and then increase the amount of time you rehearse your new role. If you are scared to try it in an actual social situation, initially begin acting it out at home alone.

It's a lot more than acting. Now get going; it's show time!

*Strictly speaking, Kelly recommended writing the sketch in the third person and describing someone you'd like to know, not someone you'd like to be. Some individuals, nevertheless, seem to get more out of the technique when it is personalized as outlined above. If one strategy doesn't work, feel free to try it the other way.

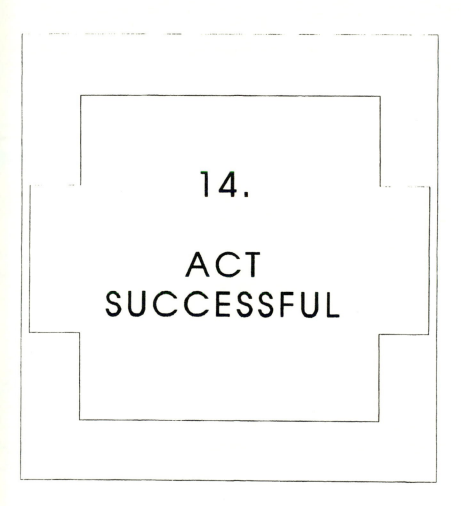

14.

ACT
SUCCESSFUL

Do you always choke up in the tenth frame of an important bowling match and toss the ball right in the old gutter? Do you always strike the "X" key when you mean to hit "A" on those timed keyboarding tests? Do you repeatedly say "USK," when you mean "USA" during public speeches?

If you answered "yes" to any of the aforementioned questions, then you owe it to yourself to try negative practice. The technique was popularized years ago by Knight Dunlap, who devoted his life to studying the making and un-making of habits.

Negative practice is simple. You merely practice making the dreadful mistake again and again and again until you become proficient at doing it wrong! (Yes, you read it correctly.)

You go out to the lanes and purposely throw numerous gutter balls. Or you give your speech in front of a mirror and keep saying "USK."

The result: When you bring the behavior under conscious control, it often will cease automatically.

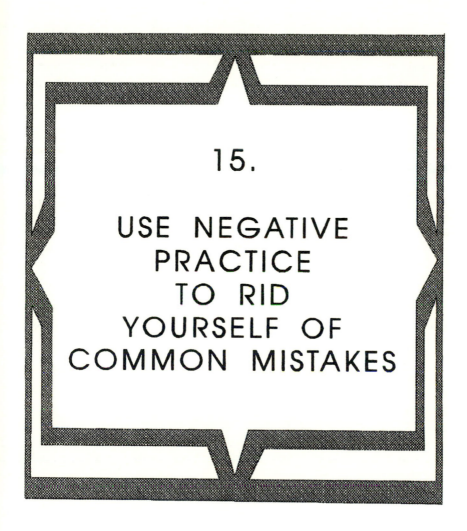

15.

USE NEGATIVE
PRACTICE
TO RID
YOURSELF OF
COMMON MISTAKES

Literally hundreds of rival schools of psychology exist. Each claims to have a stronghold on "the answer" to happiness and mental health. As you study these schools, you discover that they rarely agree on anything. The one exception is that almost all professional schools see relaxation as a beneficial activity.

How does relaxation benefit you? A better question might be, what *doesn't* it accomplish?

According to researchers, relaxation curbs tension, reduces stress, improves mood, lowers blood pressure, helps stop phobias, eliminates anxiety attacks, and even boosts the immune system.

Relaxation can be achieved in many effective ways. You can meditate. You can alternately tense and relax the major muscle groups in your body. You can turn to high-tech electronic biofeedback equipment, hypnosis, or a relaxation tape. You can imagine yourself on the beach or listen to the sounds of a bubbling brook. Or you can just sprawl out in your favorite easy chair or lawn chair.

Experiment and discover what works for you. Relax, you'll get the hang of it.

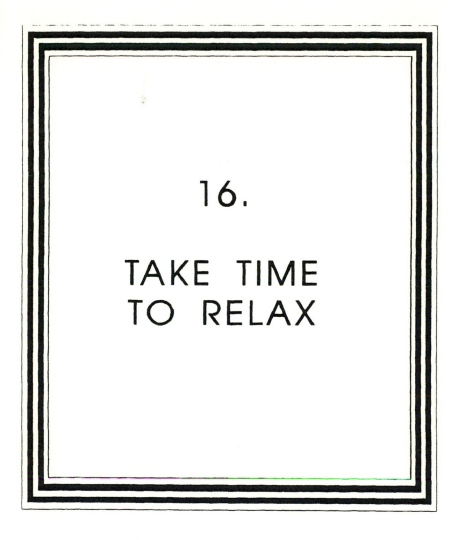

16.

TAKE TIME
TO RELAX

Happy people live; unhappy people DREAM ABOUT LIVING in the future after they experience some magical event.

Individuals who display positive mental health are doers. People who lack positive mental health are happiness procrastinators. They suffer from a mañana complex: "I won't be happy until something happens tomorrow or in the future."

Right this moment we want you to do an attitude check and discover if you have any beliefs that are prohibiting present moment happiness. Here are the types of thoughts that could be holding you back:

"I will finally be able to enjoy myself when I am married." (Interestingly enough, those who are married often say, "when I'm divorced!")

"I won't be happy until I turn 21."

"I can't really have any fun until I'm finished with law school."

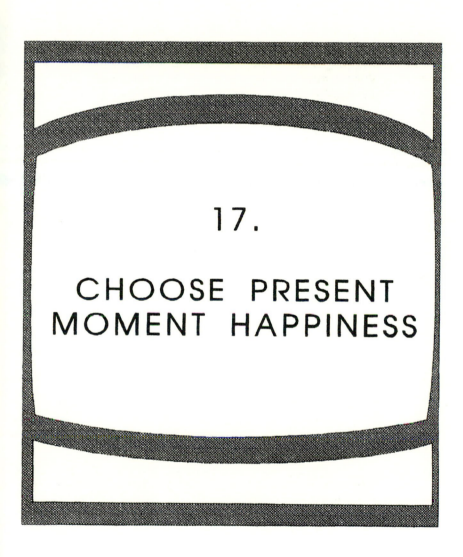

17.

CHOOSE PRESENT MOMENT HAPPINESS

Everybody experiences those so-called "days from hell" when everything goes wrong and you begin to question yourself. On days like this, you need an "emotional trophy closet" to raise your spirits.

What exactly is an emotional trophy closet? Glad you asked. An emotional trophy closet—which can be as simple as a list or an old shoe box—is a collection of successes in your life.

Your emotional trophy closet could include the following:

*A list of your positive accomplishments.

*A note your 9th-grade history teacher gave you commending your outstanding performance.

*An actual trophy you won in a golf tournament.

*A certificate you received for performing volunteer work.

*A thank you note from a friend.

Put something in your trophy closet and save it for a rainy day to make yourself feel good.

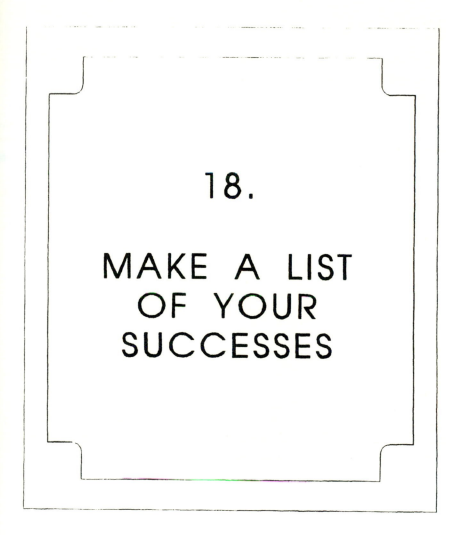

18.

MAKE A LIST
OF YOUR
SUCCESSES

Think back to the last time you had a squabble, disagreement, or an argument of barroom brawl proportions with somebody you know. The chances are excellent that you inadvertently instituted the problem or made the difficulty worse by using "you statements."

Here are some typical argument provoking "you statements":

"You hurt my feelings."

"You're responsible for my lack of confidence."

"You always make me feel inferior."

Instead of turning to "you statements," try taking responsibility for your own feelings by using this "I statement" paradigm. It goes like this: "I feel_____, when you_____, because_____. I would like_____." For example, "I feel **bad**, when you **accuse me of making too much noise**, because **I want to do things right**. I would like **to be your friend**."

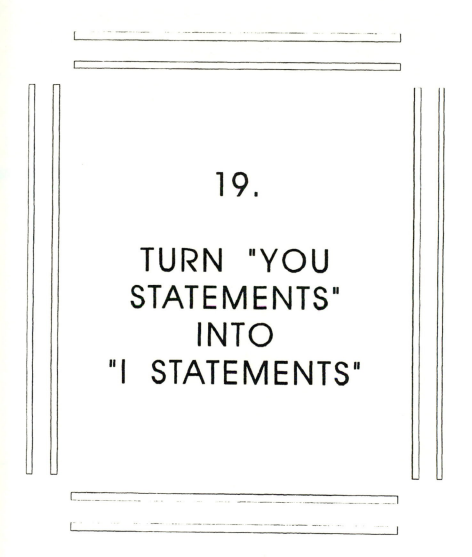

19.

TURN "YOU STATEMENTS" INTO "I STATEMENTS"

For the last 13 years, Sam has prided himself on the fact that he has bought his wife the most expensive imported chocolates money can buy for her birthday. Mary—who gets silver dollar sized welts on her face whenever she gets in striking distance of a chocolate bar—has been giving her candy to the folks at the office for (you guessed it) the last 13 years!

Mary then lets her steam out at the office as she tells her fellow workers, "I can't believe that nogoodnik Sam had the nerve to give me chocolates again this year."

Both Sam and Mary are suffering from the affliction of attempting to or expecting another to mind read.

Positive mental health is nearly impossible when you make assumptions about others. The solution is simple. Ask; don't assume anything.

Try this exercise. Pick a partner. Make an assumption about your partner (e.g., "I bet you're wearing earrings with fish on them because you have an aquarium at home.") Then have your partner respond to your assumption by explaining whether it is true or false. You'll see how mind reading can get you in trouble...and fast.

When you hear people say, "I shouldn't have to tell him; he should know I don't like so-and-so...," you're listening to a person who believes others are mind readers.

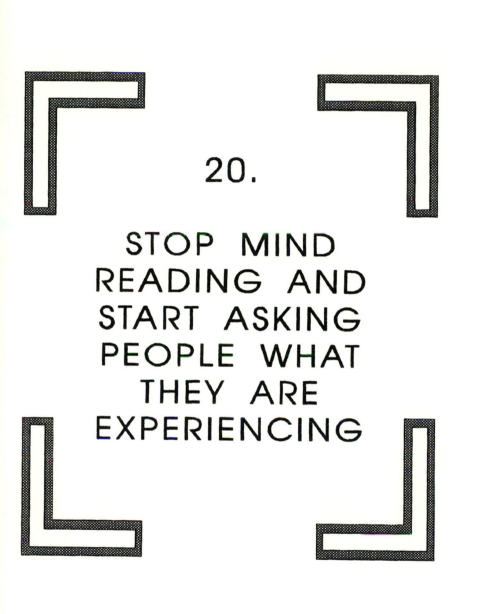

20.

STOP MIND READING AND START ASKING PEOPLE WHAT THEY ARE EXPERIENCING

Please don't ignore this wonderful little technique just because it's so easy to use. If you have a behavior you want to reduce or eliminate, such as nail biting or smoking, make a chart of the behavior.

The mere act of charting the behavior is a chore and, therefore, often makes it more difficult to engage in the behavior. Hence, the incidence of the behavior is often reduced.

It doesn't matter what the chart looks like as long as it makes sense to you.

Best of all, charting can be combined with other strategies you decide to implement.

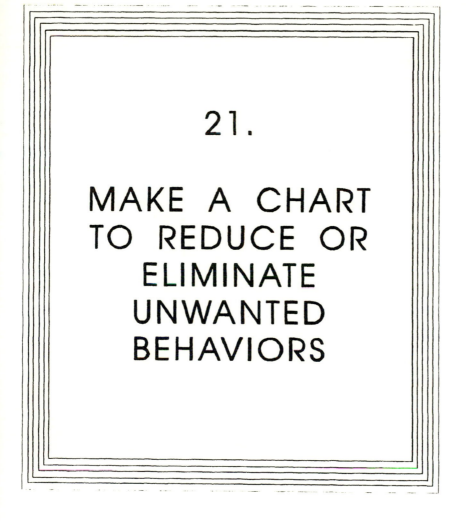

21.

MAKE A CHART TO REDUCE OR ELIMINATE UNWANTED BEHAVIORS

Cursing was becoming commonplace in the office, and some people weren't taking kindly to it. A cuss jar was thus placed in the center of the work area. Each foul word was assigned a "cost," from 25 cents to (gulp!) $2.00. Every time an employee uttered a no-no word, the other employees made sure the proper amount was placed in the jar.

Now here's the kicker. At the end of the month, the money in the jar was donated to a cause that everybody in the office OPPOSED!

The result: A curse-free office in less than 14 days!

Now cost doesn't have to involve money. Parents often discover that removing children's privileges, for example, seems to work rather well.

So if you want to engage in the self-defeating behavior...well go right ahead. But remember, this time around it's going to cost you!

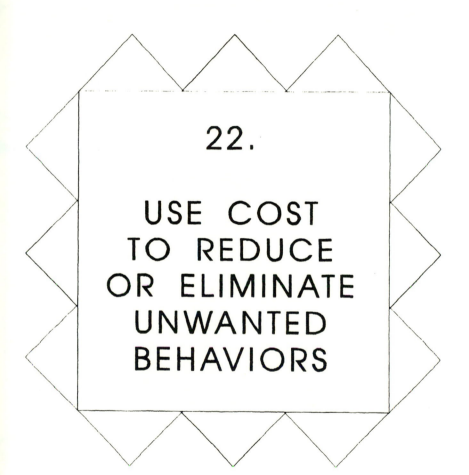

22.

**USE COST
TO REDUCE
OR ELIMINATE
UNWANTED
BEHAVIORS**

Behavioral scientists technically refer to this process as "reframing." You can, for example, look at a single glass of water and see it as "half empty," or positively relabel it as "half full."

Similarly, you can look in the mirror and mumble something about getting old, or you can smile at yourself and praise how distinguished you look.

You can catastrophize about the horrendous, boring time you must spend alone, or you can relabel it and look forward to that special time when you can relax and catch up on your reading.

Make a list of things in your life that need relabeling. Then try out some new labels associated with positive emotions and watch how much brighter your life seems.

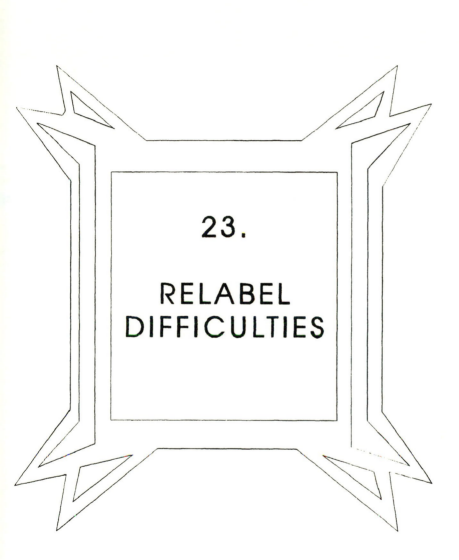

23.

RELABEL
DIFFICULTIES

Ben never looked forward to the holidays. He felt they were too materialistic and commercialized. Nevertheless, last year he volunteered his time at a food bank, and he felt great.

Do something for somebody else. Not only will it take your mind off your troubles, but you'll be performing a valuable service.

The royal road to helping yourself often begins with helping others.

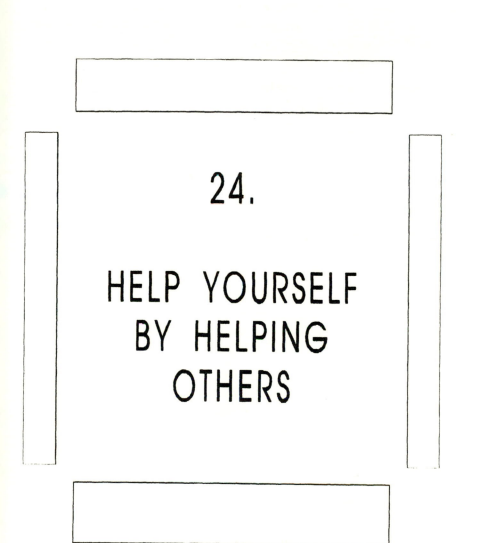

24.

HELP YOURSELF BY HELPING OTHERS

Mr. Hensen has been giving his college math class the same assignments for over 10 years. Mrs. Dickson always vacations at the same resort. Ms. York has been performing the same exercise routine faithfully since her second son was born. Her son is now a senior at Harvard.

Mr. Hensen tells the other college professors that he's tired of teaching math, though he doesn't have a clue why. Mrs. Dickson confides in a neighbor that she doesn't understand it but she no longer looks forward to vacations. And last but not least, poor Ms. York is baffled that her exercise routine just doesn't yield results like it did "in the late 60s."

Now granted, there is something to be said for stability and life's everyday routines. Nevertheless, when each day is NEARLY IDENTICAL to the day that came before it and the day that is coming after it, life becomes mundane, depressing, and downright boring!

The solution...creativity. Do something different. When you wake up, you'll have something new and exciting to look forward to.

Some ways to implement this might include the following:

* Drive home from work using a different route.
* Eat a new food.
* Go to a lecture on a subject you know nothing about.
* Read a book you normally would never read.
* Try a new hairstyle or mode of dress.

So fight boredom. Carry a note card with you that says: **"A new day, a new way.**

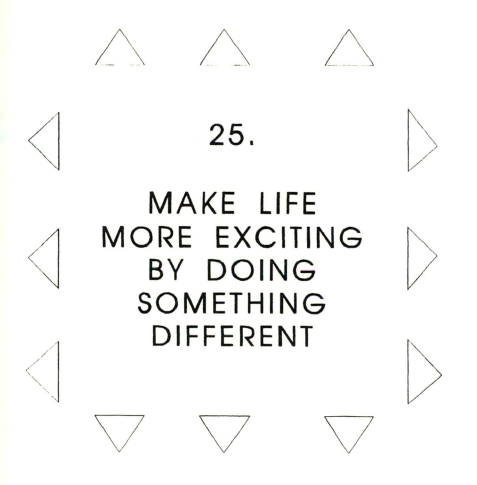

25.

MAKE LIFE MORE EXCITING BY DOING SOMETHING DIFFERENT

Mandy currently attends an accelerated private high school. The admission requirements are tough. Each student must possess a near genius IQ. Since Mandy's IQ was extremely high, the school ACCEPTED HER WITH OPEN ARMS. By a strange twist of events, Mandy's mother discovered that Mandy's test score had been switched with another student's who had a similar last name! Much to her mother's chagrin, Mandy's actual score indicated her intelligence was at best "just average."

According to the test, Mandy should have been struggling, making poor grades, or more likely flunking out.

So what precisely was happening in Mandy's academic career? The answer is easy. Because of her FIRM CONVICTION that she was a genius, she led the class with straight A's, three years running!

In a landmark experiment, individuals who were allergic to a given leaf were touched with a harmless leaf but were told it was one that triggered the allergy. The result? Most of the individuals immediately experienced a severe allergic reaction! Next the subjects were touched with the culprit (the leaf that truly produced the allergy) but were told it was harmless. Of course, you can guess what transpired. The subjects—BELIEVING the leaf was harmless—experienced no reaction whatsoever!!!

There's a popular saying among hypnotists: If you believe you can, you're right; you can. If you believe you can't, you're right; you can't.

The point is simple. Stop waiting for an IQ test, a parent, a boyfriend, a girlfriend, a baker, a candlestick maker, or some board certified expert to confirm or disprove your "ok-ness." Instead, BELIEVE in yourself. Only you can do it...and you CAN DO IT!

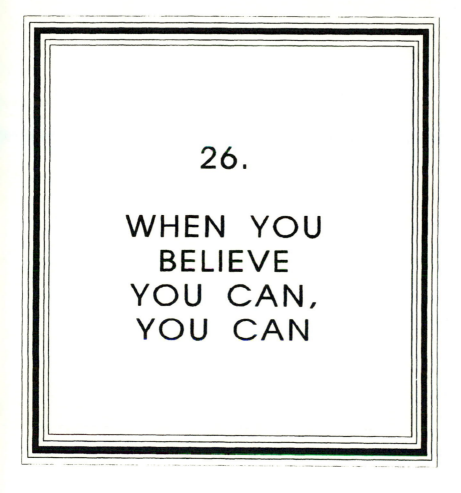

26.

WHEN YOU
BELIEVE
YOU CAN,
YOU CAN

Do you have clay on your feet? That's right clay—excess baggage and fear from your past that is keeping you from being a happy, successful, creative person? Examples are thoughts such as

"I always get rejected, so I steer clear of relationships."

"I always finish last, so why try."

"I'm a Johnson, and the Johnsons always avoided change."

"I've always been afraid to take action."

Note the word "always" and how it can often hold you back. Remember that the past is not the present, and it certainly isn't the future.

So shake the clay away and try walking from this point on with clean feet. Wipe the slate clean. Start with a new beginning. Forget about what has "always happened before."

How do you know when you've accomplished this? That's easy. For the first time you'll be able to look down and actually see your toes and your ankles.

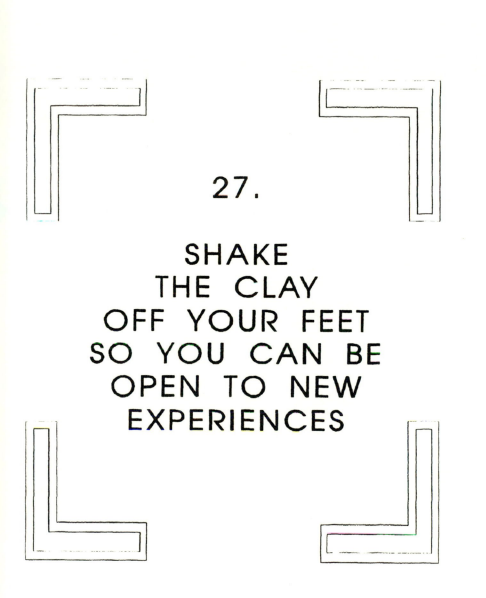

27.

SHAKE
THE CLAY
OFF YOUR FEET
SO YOU CAN BE
OPEN TO NEW
EXPERIENCES

Wait. Yes, that's your alarm clock. And yes, it's time to get up...but don't move a muscle until you come up with something you can do to raise your spirits. Positive mental health takes a little bit of planning, you know.

Please, give it some thought. This is serious and you need to put some energy into this task. (At least as much energy as you're putting into the question, "What's for breakfast?")

You merely ask yourself, "What can I do today so I'll feel better about myself?"

"But that's so simple," you say. Well if it's so simple, then why aren't you doing it?

Just imagine how good you would feel at the end of one week if you just did one small thing each day to boost your morale.

So the choice is really yours. Seven days from now you can still be dreaming about feeling better, or you can make just one change per day and ride the road to positive mental health. You decide!

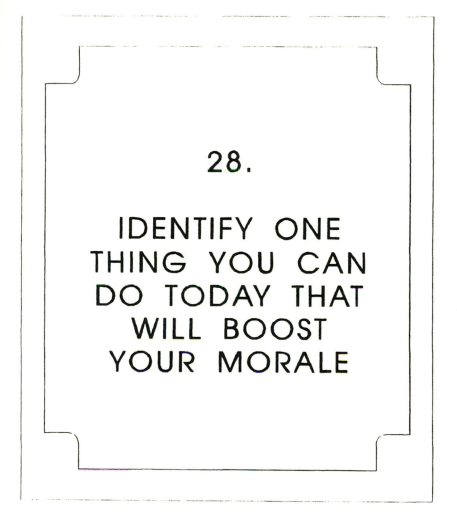

28.

IDENTIFY ONE THING YOU CAN DO TODAY THAT WILL BOOST YOUR MORALE

Do you know how severely depressed people think? Psychologists and professional counselors do. They call it "dichotomous thinking." It's either/or logic. For example:

"Either I get this raise, or I'll never ask for another one again."

"Either I get a straight A report card, or my academic career is over."

"Either Beth goes to the prom with me, or I swear I'll never date another woman again."

"Either I get this job, or I'll kill myself." (Just imagine if everybody thought this way and there were 500 applicants! One-half of the city's population could be wiped out!)

THINKING LIKE THIS IS ENOUGH TO DEPRESS ANYBODY! GIVE IT UP NOW AND YOU'LL NEVER REGRET IT! Look for other options. In most cases, there are more than two extreme positions.

To rid yourself of this tendency, it is best to force yourself to make a list of other viable alternatives.

If, for example, Beth doesn't go to the prom with you, why not tag along with your younger brother to the auto show? Perhaps you'll meet the woman of your dreams. Or you could ask Rachel to go to the prom with you. You've always wondered if she was more your type anyway. And so on...

Stop basing your life on the outcome of a single event...it's not helping you and it's certainly unfair to the other 499 job applicants!

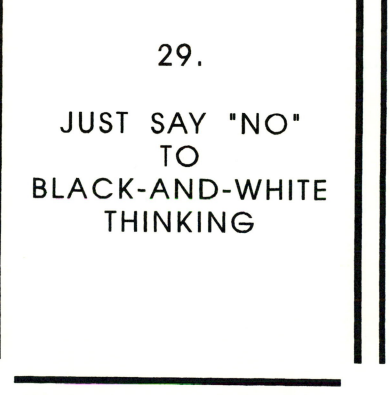

29.

JUST SAY "NO"
TO
BLACK-AND-WHITE
THINKING

Dan always thought of himself as tough. Everybody knows, a macho dude like him would never express feelings of sadness. That would be a sign of unmanliness.

Dan always felt he could handle anything on his own. When he was a youngster, it was drilled into his head that only "weak" or "crazy" people ask for help. He was taught to keep a stiff upper lip and deal with difficulties on his own.

His best friend Fred, nevertheless, could see that, since Dan's breakup with Linda, he was depressed and going downhill fast. Fred insisted that Dan visit a counselor at least once. Although Dan didn't believe in "publicly airing his dirty laundry" (a line he heard a thousand times growing up), he agreed to see the counselor one time to PROVE it wouldn't help.

After the session, Dan was surprised (perhaps shocked would be a better word) to discover that HE DID FEEL BETTER. He had, in fact, agreed eagerly to see the counselor again next week and actually was looking forward to his next session!

Dan's experience was not atypical. Counselors see it almost daily. So, if you're hurting and feelings are building up inside of you, find a caring friend you can trust and talk about it.

If that doesn't help, seek out a qualified professional (e.g., a school counselor, therapist, or psychologist). Your local mental health association, crisis hotline, or hospital can give you some resources.

Just talking about your feelings helps. Experts call it "catharsis."

So, to the Dans of the world, listen up: Take a small risk and discover that there really is a talking cure.

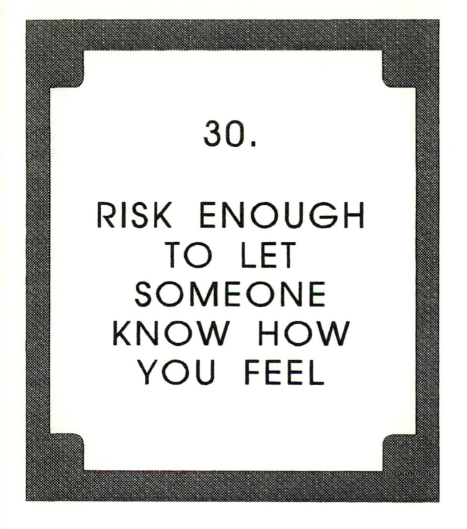

30.

RISK ENOUGH
TO LET
SOMEONE
KNOW HOW
YOU FEEL

A number of years ago, behavioral scientists discovered an amazing, novel, high-tech form of behavior therapy called "biofeedback." By being hooked up to a sophisticated electronic device that revealed biological feedback, an individual could learn to change his or her behavior.

When a person could see or hear his biological reaction, then the person could learn to control his heart rate, muscle tension, hand temperature, and even brain waves! It was considered remarkable—a true scientific breakthrough.

Well, if you lean forward and come a little closer, I'll tell you a little secret. No, make that a big secret. Unbeknownst to you, you already have a biofeedback device in your home. Yes. Honest, I'm leveling with you. In fact, YOUR biofeedback device yields more information than any of the expensive computerized units. It's called a mirror!

Now go to your mirror, put on a mile-wide smile and take a good long look at yourself. Isn't that the way you want to look and feel? Fine, then spend a few minutes in front of the mirror each day and get in touch with the pleasant, joyful side of your personality. Get some biofeedback. Practice makes perfect.

Stop being so serious...the guy or girl in the mirror isn't.

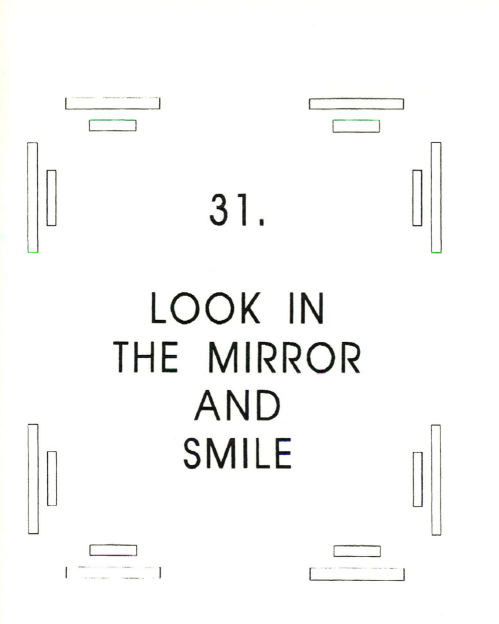

31.

LOOK IN
THE MIRROR
AND
SMILE

Mr. Dixon was furious over the critical remarks his boss made. Rather than deal with his feelings, he suppressed them using denial. On his way home, he honked and cursed at other drivers, and drove in a manner that could only be described as dangerous and reckless.

The moment he walked in the door he began yelling at his wife and four-year-old daughter.

"But, Daddy, I didn't do anything," protested Mr. Dixon's daughter. Yes, in this case, wisdom really did emanate from the mouth of a babe.

Mr. Dixon's daughter is, of course, correct. She didn't do anything wrong. Her father is a victim of displaced anger.

Mr. Dixon's first step is to be honest with himself and acknowledge his feelings. Of course it's scary, but it's a necessary step in the quest for positive mental health.

And the second step...is carefully outlined in the next strategy for positive mental health. You'll discover it by turning to the next page.

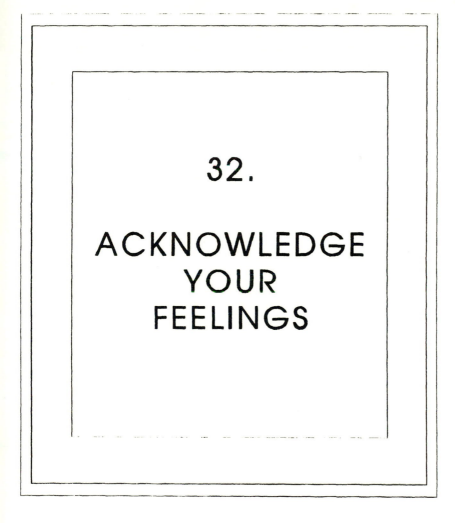

32.

ACKNOWLEDGE YOUR FEELINGS

Expressing your feelings constructively does not mean kicking in the living room door or punching a hole in the bedroom wall. It does not mean driving like an insane maniac or giving other drivers obscene gestures. And it certainly doesn't mean (and Mr. Dixon from the last example, we hope YOU'RE reading this) yelling at your wife and screaming at your poor daughter when you're really ticked off at your boss!

Try to tell the person whom you believe is responsible for your feelings (1) how you feel, (2) why you think you feel that way, and (3) what you would like him or her to do differently.

Sure it's a lot easier, and often psychologically safer, to take your feelings out on a door, a wall, an unknown driver, your family pet, or your four-old-daughter (after all, your boss can fire you; your four-year-old daughter can't); but how will these actions help you solve the difficulty?

Keep in mind that for some folks positive feelings are just as difficult to express as negative ones. When positive feelings are not ventilated openly, friends and lovers often go their separate ways. BE POSITIVE...AND DON'T LET IT HAPPEN TO YOU!

P.S. Mr. Dixon, do the world a favor and let your boss know how you feel!

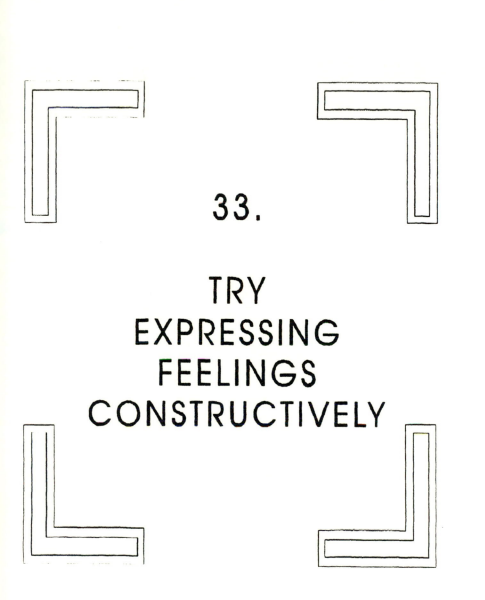

33.

TRY
EXPRESSING
FEELINGS
CONSTRUCTIVELY

Some folks rush from project to project so rapidly that if they blink, they'll miss it. The problem with this philosophy of life is that these individuals never get to savor the moment and enjoy a job well done.

When you complete a task, try taking a little time out to practice self-appreciation. Stand back. Look at what you've accomplished. Nice job, isn't it? Okay, then let's cut the self-modesty bit and give yourself a pat on the back. You deserve it.

If it feels a bit odd just remind yourself, you earned it!

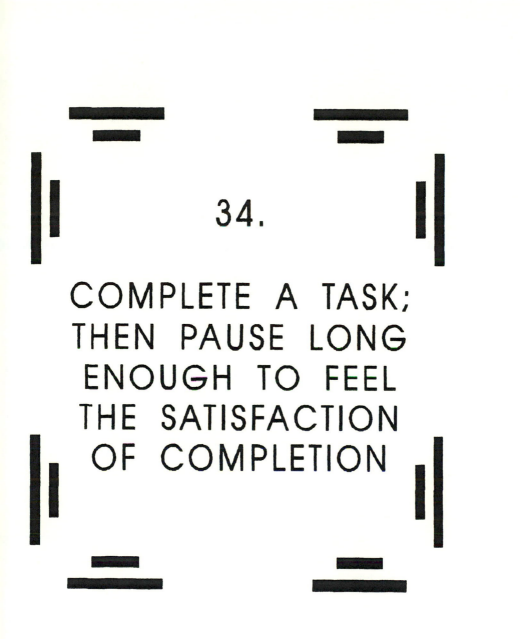

34.

COMPLETE A TASK; THEN PAUSE LONG ENOUGH TO FEEL THE SATISFACTION OF COMPLETION

Christy was furious. She had her hair permed, colored, and completely restyled, yet her best friend, Allison, didn't even notice.

"I just hate her; she's so self-centered," Christy told her roommate. "All Allison cares about is herself. I could care less if I never see her again."

Whoa there, Christy! Slow down and learn to practice what behavioral scientists call "accurate empathy."

Empathy is the act of trying to understand the feelings and actions of another person "as if" you ARE that person.

Did you know, Christy, that Allison's grandmother was rushed to the hospital emergency room last night and is still in intensive care? Were you aware that her basement was flooded and many of her family heirlooms were ruined? And did you know that her sciatica is killing her (ouch!!!) even though she's living on prescription pain pills?

Oh, you didn't know. That's what I thought.

Well, here. Slip this pair of Allison's moccasins on and see if hairstyles come to mind.

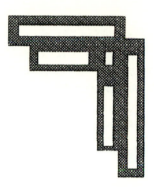
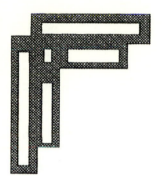

35.

BEFORE YOU JUDGE SOMEONE ELSE, TAKE A WALK IN HIS OR HER SHOES

Mr. Dennison had spent 13 hard years struggling to become the chief executive officer of his company. He now has a six-figure income, a rare imported sports car, and two summer vacation homes. When he's at work, he spends most of his time at business meetings making decisions in the world of high finance.

There is only one problem. Mr. Dennison is unhappy...very unhappy.

In a rare moment, when Mr. Dennison was totally honest with himself, he closed his eyes and tried to reflect on who he really was. He decided that he couldn't have cared less about his job, and the material goods he had amassed, including his vacation homes.

These things might please somebody else. They were indeed indicative of success in our society, but THEY WEREN'T A PART OF HIS "REAL ME."

Mr. Dennison's "real me" was a farmer living outside a small town. His imported sports car ideally would be replaced with a dust covered pickup truck and an old tractor. Instead of his vacation houses he would have a barn.

Now close your eyes and have a look. The "REAL ME" is just waiting to come out and take a peek.

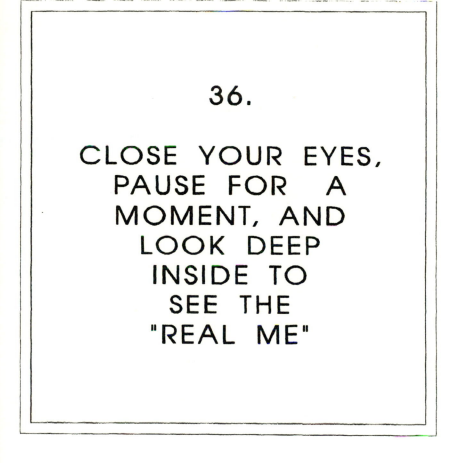

36.

CLOSE YOUR EYES,
PAUSE FOR A
MOMENT, AND
LOOK DEEP
INSIDE TO
SEE THE
"REAL ME"

The best way to handle a fearful situation is to DO SOMETHING ABOUT IT!

Experts often recommend a program called "in vivo desensitization." It is very effective even if you have difficulty pronouncing the term!

The secret of in vivo desensitization is to confront the fear very, very slowly...to creep up on it, if you will. So...

If you turn pink at the thought of riding an elevator, begin by spending a few minutes a day standing next to the elevator. Keep doing this until you can remain relaxed. Polish your nails on a bench in front of one, or perhaps chow down on a baloney sandwich while you calmly size the elevator up. Next...

Spend a few days walking up to the elevator and pushing the button...just pushing the button...you're not riding anywhere yet! Then...

Walk onto the elevator and push the pause button. Spend a little time in the elevator; get to know it a little better. Finally, when the elevator seems a tad friendlier...

Ride the elevator with a friend a few times. Then hop in it again and ride it with your friend nearby. You could discover that you really enjoy riding the elevator.

Be creative. Be calm. Move slowly. Creep up on your fears. You can do it. The only thing you have to fear is not taking action!

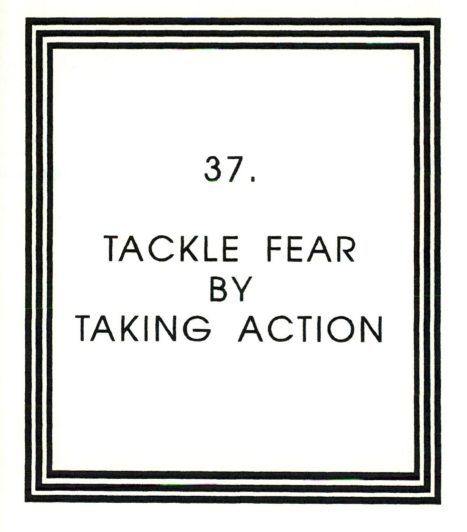

37.

TACKLE FEAR
BY
TAKING ACTION

The world can be a cruel place. If you don't believe it, try watching the national news. War, crime, poverty, illness, prejudice, and natural disasters are featured daily.

The good news (no pun intended) is that you—yes you—can pitch in and make the world a better place. How? Well you can begin by smiling at someone you don't know.

You don't need to be a rocket scientist to figure out that when you frown at somebody, the person often feels bad. The person might ask, "I wonder what is wrong with me?"

Smiling, however, generally elicits the opposite response. The person feels accepted.

Oh come on now. Don't say you can't do it. If a six-week-old baby can do it, you can too!

38.

SHARE A SMILE
WITH SOMEONE
YOU DON'T
KNOW

Have you ever been in a situation with several alternatives and were unsure which course of action you needed to take? Some examples are

"Should I take out the trash? Of course, I'm supposed to, but my parents won't know the difference; they're out of town."

"Should I yell at the store clerk? After all, I definitely was treated unfairly."

"Should I offer to help that gentleman carry his groceries? He seems to have more than he can handle."

And so on...

David reported that as a young child his dad showed him how to stick a banana into the exhaust pipe of a police car. Yesterday David—who is now 22—was arrested for doing the same thing!!!

Here's a terrific little technique. Just imagine that somebody is watching you. Say a young child is watching you, and that child is going to watch your behavior and then IMITATE it. So you ask yourself, "Is this what I want that child (or anyone else for that matter!) to do?"

A theory of behavior known as "social learning theory" clearly indicates that others will mimic our behavior. YOUR JOB IS TO GIVE OTHERS THE BEST BEHAVIOR TO MIMIC! You'll be helping others, you'll sleep a lot better, and we guarantee you'll have a lot more bananas to eat! Think about it.

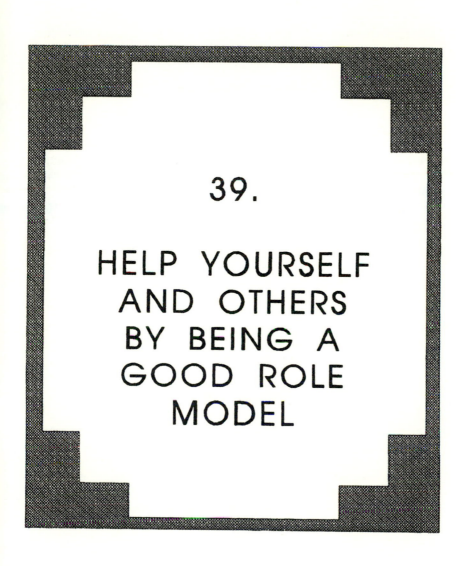

39.

HELP YOURSELF
AND OTHERS
BY BEING A
GOOD ROLE
MODEL

Millie's father died, and she never told him how much she loved him. Barry's girlfriend of four years dumped him, yet he could never ventilate his intense anger. Leslie's deceased father sexually abused her, yet she was unable to confront him while he was alive.

Millie, Barry, and Leslie all would benefit by writing a FEELING letter. Here's how it's done. You write a letter using lots of statements beginning with "I feel."

When you write the letter, you must write it and rewrite until you do your feelings justice. Don't hold back. Be totally frank and brutally honest. Sugarcoat nothing! Give it to the person straight, and don't pull any punches. LET IT ALL HANG OUT!

When your letter is completed, read it out loud. Then put it away for a week or so and see how you feel. If your feelings are still pushing on your insides like a balloon ready to explode, you'll need to add additional feelings or edit the work.

There is NO NEED TO SEND THE LETTER (and needless to say, in the case of a deceased person, it would be downright impossible). It is often helpful to read what you have written to others whom you can trust, such as members of a counseling group.

So if you can lick a stamp, you can lick your problem. On second thought, save the licks for an ice cream celebration.

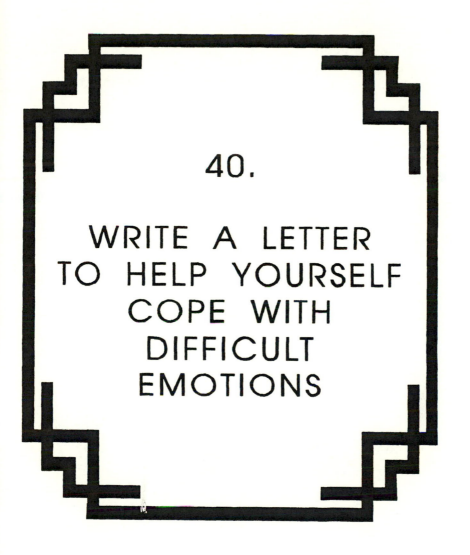

40.

WRITE A LETTER TO HELP YOURSELF COPE WITH DIFFICULT EMOTIONS

In a famous experiment dubbed as "Pygmalion in the Classroom," teachers were told that certain grade school pupils had taken intelligence tests and were "late bloomers" who would show profound improvement during the school year. In reality, these were just plain ordinary students picked at random. The students were unaware that the teachers were told anything.

Intelligence tests administered at the end of the academic year indicated that the "bloomers" did improve more than the other children. They had higher grades and amazingly enough, even higher IQ scores!

THE TEACHERS EXPECTED THESE CHILDREN TO DO WELL, AND THEY DID!!!

Most likely, the teachers—because of their conviction that these students were some pretty smart cookies—unconsciously treated these students in a manner that was conducive to their growth and improvement.

Behavioral scientists sometimes refer to this phenomenon as a "self-fulfilling prophecy."

Now examine yourself. Are you giving others the benefit of the doubt? Are you looking for the positive qualities in people or do you focus on the negative? Well?

Start looking for the good in others...because the best way to make yourself blossom is to help others bloom.

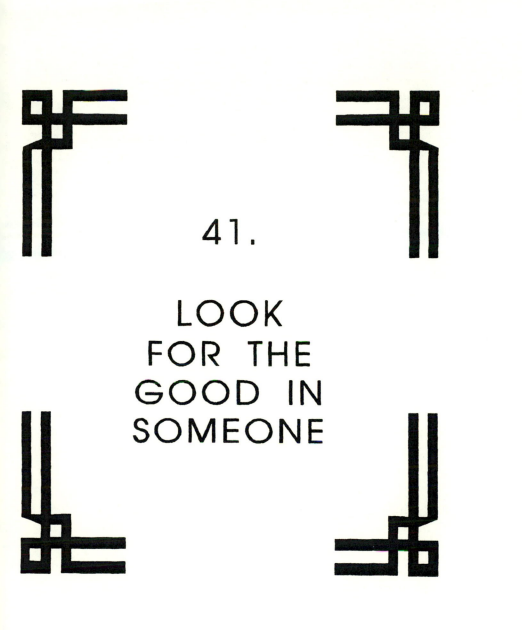

41.

LOOK
FOR THE
GOOD IN
SOMEONE

It's 7 a.m., and Lance is awakened by his alarm clock. At 8:30, Lance is scheduled to attend his History 101 class at Tegner Community College. As he shaves, his thoughts race.

"I hate getting up early. College is so stupid. Who gives a hoot about history?...I sure as heck don't. And I have to fight that stupid traffic on Highway 9 again. Another lousy day, I wish it was over already."

An interesting perspective. It's 7:02 in the morning, and Lance has already convinced himself he's going to have a crummy day.

However...

It's 7 a.m., and Kelly is awakened by her alarm clock. At 8:30, Kelly is scheduled to attend her History 101 class at Tegner Community College. As she puts on her make-up, her thoughts race.

"I love getting up early. That way I don't feel like I'm missing an important part of the day. College is terrific, especially that History 101 class. Great stuff! Who knows, perhaps I'll major in history and become an elementary teacher...or...or...I could use what I'm learning if I ever write a novel. Oh yes! And the trees on Highway 9 are just beautiful this time of year. It's a great day! I might even see that really cute guy Lance in class."

An interesting perspective. It's 7:02 in the morning, and Kelly already has convinced herself she's going to have a wonderful day.

There's a saying among sanitation engineers that sums it up quite nicely: Garbage in—garbage out.

Perhaps it's time for you to take out the garbage. Set your alarm and sleep on it.

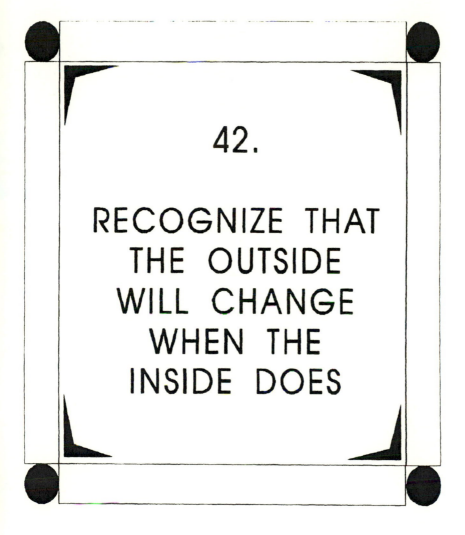

42.

RECOGNIZE THAT THE OUTSIDE WILL CHANGE WHEN THE INSIDE DOES

Most people hopelessly practice the "more-of-the-same-habit." Unfortunately, the more-of-the-same-habit is about as useful as a bicycle with flat tires, though the more-of-the-same-habit is plagued with a little more hot air.

To comprehend precisely how the more-of-the-same-habit undermines our happiness, let's look at the case of Paul.

Paul's little sister is constantly sneaking in his room to take his CDs and cassette tapes. Each time she does this, he screams at her loud enough to shake the bedroom windows. It has happened about 50 or 60 times...and Paul (who is now hoarse) is still screaming at her. The problem is SHE'S STILL DOING IT!

So take a hint, Paul: Your screaming and carrying on isn't doing one bit of good. If this strategy was working, your sister would have stopped taking your music after a very short period of time.

THE MORAL OF THE STORY IS CLEARLY THAT IF SOMETHING ISN'T WORKING, GIVE IT UP AND TRY SOMETHING DIFFERENT!

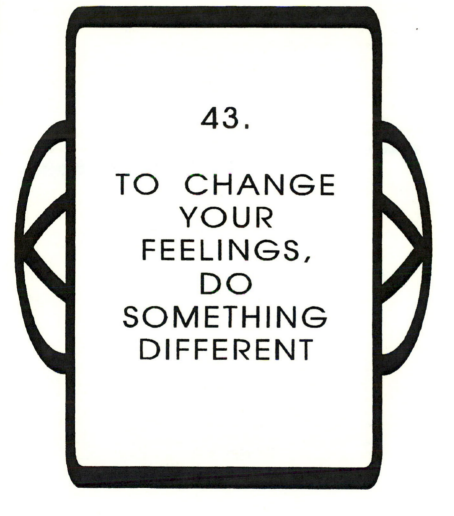

43.

TO CHANGE
YOUR
FEELINGS,
DO
SOMETHING
DIFFERENT

If life hands you a bowl of prune pits when you expected a bowl of cherries, then it's time to turn to the five-step problem-solving method.

Okay. First, think of a really tough problem. You thought of one...terrific. Now number a sheet of paper from 1 to 5, leaving a few spaces to write between each number.

Here are the five steps: 1. Define the difficulty. 2. List your options. 3. Create a plan. 4. Implement the plan. 5. Evaluate your efforts.

Let's go through a trial run:

1. DEFINE: "I'm totally worthless." (Sorry, but you need to be specific and define the problem in terms of your behavior.) "Um...let's see...I feel worthless because I'm unemployed." (Now you've got the hang of it).

2. OPTIONS: "Utilize the services of an employment office; see a professional career counselor; look for jobs in the newspaper; tell everyone I know that I'm looking for work; stop thinking of myself as worthless." (Say, you really DO have a lot of options.)

3. PLAN: "On Monday, visit the state employment office; on Tuesday, set up an appointment to see the career counselor at the school I graduated from; on Wednesday, obtain a daily paper, read the help wanted ads, and respond to those appropriate; on Thursday, telephone everybody in my address book; on Friday, contact a therapist to help rid me of my stinkin' thinkin'. After all, it doesn't mean I'm worthless just because I'm unemployed."

4. IMPLEMENT: "Get off my duff and DO what I said I'd do in my plan." (Good point. The best plan in the world is useless if it's never implemented.)

5. EVALUATE: "Look, I'm getting a paycheck now and I'm feeling pretty good about myself; can't we go to the next postive mental health strategy?"

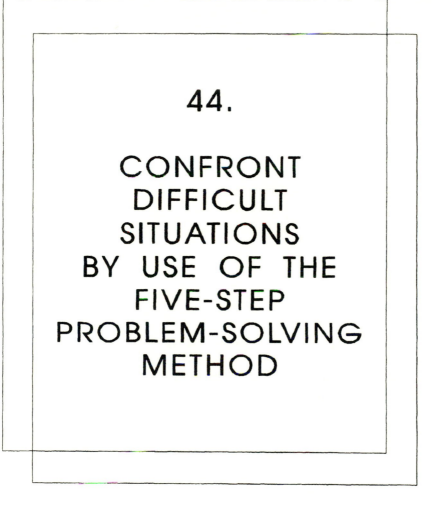

44.

CONFRONT DIFFICULT SITUATIONS BY USE OF THE FIVE-STEP PROBLEM-SOLVING METHOD

JIM: "I can't believe you ran the credit card up to more than $3,000 again!"

CHERYL: "Me? Me? You've got to be out of your mind!"

JIM: "Yes, you! Who do you think ran it up, Skippy our pet gerbil?"

CHERYL: "Oh, yes, I almost forgot...mister genius here. We're the only couple in town that owns a gerbil with a dog's name. Brilliant name, Jimmy, very creative."

JIM: "Stop being sarcastic and quit trying to change the subject; we've got a credit card the size of Mount Everest!"

CHERYL: "Of course we do sweetheart. That usually happens when you buy golf clubs and useless power tools that sell for more than a small battleship!"

FOLKS, PLEASE...TIME OUT!

As you can see, this argument is going nowhere fast; in fact, it's going nowhere PERIOD. You see, Cheryl and Jim (whether they know it or not) have something in common: Both are 101% convinced that their own stance is the correct one.

Here's what needs to happen next. Cheryl and Jim need to continue the argument EXCEPT THAT JIM SHOULD ARGUE AS IF HE IS CHERYL, AND CHERYL SHOULD FORCE HERSELF TO ARGUE AS IF SHE IS JIM.

Try it sometime. You could BOTH discover that the other person has a good point.

45.

USE ROLE REVERSAL TO TAKE THE STING OUT OF A NASTY ARGUMENT

After Harry met Sally at the office, each became head-over-heels in love with the other. Harry, however, never told Sally how he felt. Sally, likewise, never expressed her feelings for Harry.

Today is the day of the company picnic. Harry is home watching the baseball game on television. This is the only way he knows how to cope with his loneliness. Sally is sitting in her apartment wringing out her crying towel. She wonders if she will ever find a man who cares enough about her to date her on a regular basis.

Please don't complicate the issue:

If you like somebody, say so.

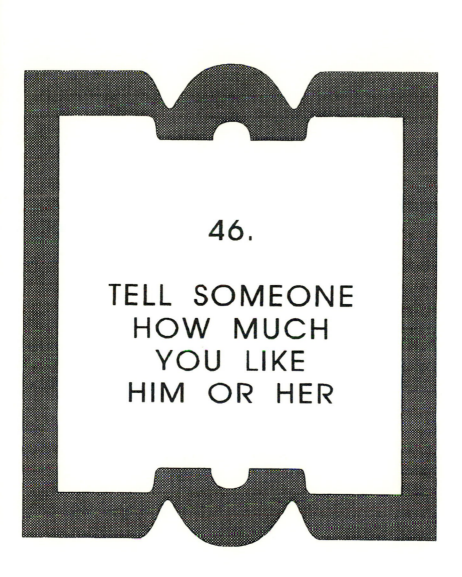

46.

TELL SOMEONE
HOW MUCH
YOU LIKE
HIM OR HER

Without a doubt, human beings are social creatures. However, when Sandy told her counselor that she had not spent an evening alone in over six months, her counselor wisely prescribed some "homework" assignments so that Sandy could become more comfortable with herself.

She was instructed to do the following:

1. Stay home and engage in a pleasurable activity such as taking a bubble bath.
2. Go to a movie alone.
3. Take a one-day trip to a city where you do not know anybody.
4. Treat yourself to a meal at a nice restaurant.
5. Go to the park alone and attempt to sketch a picture of the scenery.

The person who learns to feel comfortable alone, ends up feeling even better when he or she is around others.

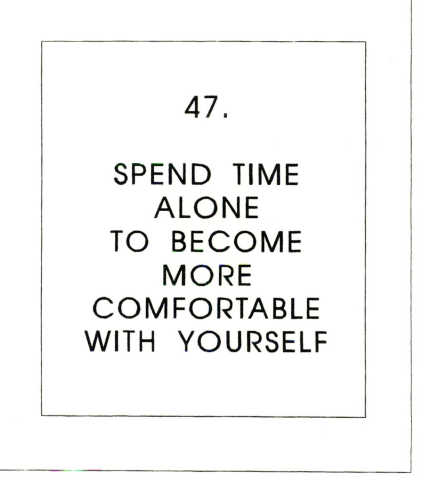

47.

SPEND TIME
ALONE
TO BECOME
MORE
COMFORTABLE
WITH YOURSELF

"There's nothing either good or bad but thinking makes it so," said Shakespeare expressing his wisdom in *Hamlet*.

Dr. Albert Ellis, a world renown clinical psychologist, has spent the better part of his career studying human misery and is thoroughly convinced that the majority of it is the result of irrational thinking.

According to Dr. Ellis, disturbance is produced in this manner:

* At A we have an activating event.

* At B we have a belief system in regards to the event.

* At C we have an emotional consequence. And, if the belief at B is irrational or illogical, then the emotional consequence at C is usually undesirable.

So what are those irrational ideas lurking in the dark shadows at point B? Here are some of the prime culprits:

1. **You feel everyone must love or approve of you.** This is irrational since it is impossible...you can't attain it!

2. **You believe unhappiness is caused by outside events and is out of your control.** Not true, points out Ellis—unhappiness comes largely from within. The Stoic philosopher, Epictetus, remarked in the first century A.D.: "Men are disturbed not by things, but by the views they take of them." Was this guy ahead of his time or what?

3. **You tell yourself it is awful when things don't go your way.** Instead ask yourself why things should be different? Moreover, awfulizing makes the situation seem even worse.

4. **You believe the past determines your present behavior, and, thus, you cannot change the way you feel.** Although it may be difficult, you can force yourself to act and think differently in the present.

5. **You think it is easier to run away from life's difficulties than to face them.** Wrong! Avoiding something leads to a lack of self-confidence.

IF YOU WANT POSITIVE MENTAL HEALTH, YOU'LL NEED TO MOVE ON TO D...WORKING AS HARD AS YOU CAN TO **DISPUTE** THESE IDEAS! It's only rational, you know.

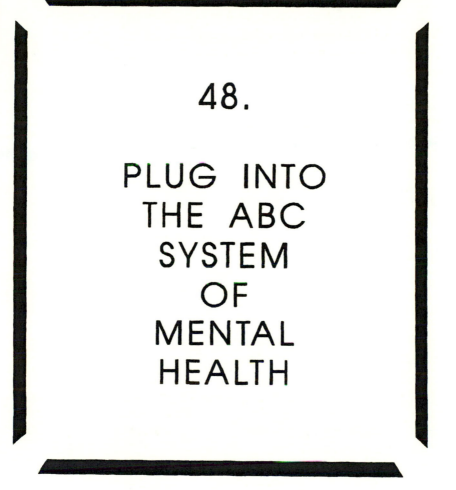

48.

PLUG INTO THE ABC SYSTEM OF MENTAL HEALTH

Imagine going to see a movie at Anywhere USA. It's your basic psychological thriller. Here is what you'll most likely see.

The main character has lived with a morbid fear of dogs for as long as he can remember. In an attempt to discover why, the star of the silver screen will spend three gruelling years, four days a week, no less, unravelling the complexities of his childhood with his dedicated analyst. Finally, one day during a landmark session, he uncovers THE REASON for his problem.

At the tender age of 3 1/2 years, he had been attacked viciously on his back porch by an irate doberman. The memory was so painful he automatically forgot about the whole incident. His psychoanalyst will call this phenomenon "repression."

When the repression is lifted, the patient has insight—knowledge of what is really causing the present difficulty—and he will be cured.

At that point our hero will ride off into the sunset and live happily ever after. (Until we see him again in his next blockbuster movie.)

Now true to life, SOME PEOPLE, SOME OF THE TIME, ARE CURED IN PRECISELY THIS MANNER. Sadly enough, others spend their entire lives searching for THE TRUTH, hopping from therapist to therapist and never find the answer. Others attain insight—discover THE REASON FOR THEIR DIFFICULTY—and STILL behave in the same manner!

The moral of the story, or shall we say the movie, is that you should do everything in your power to try to change NOW! Don't wait for a magic memory to appear—first, because it may never happen, and second, because it may not alter the situation anyway.

Insight is good if you can get it, but it's not always necessary. Make a decision—yes, right this very minute—to change NOW!

This method won't sell a lot of rush-hour tickets, popcorn, or soda, but it sure beats the long lines at the insight show.

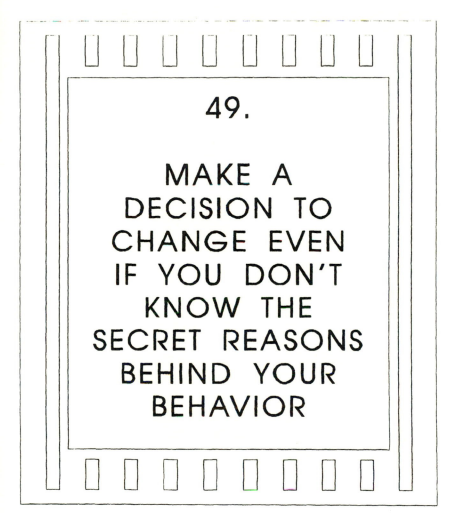

49.

MAKE A DECISION TO CHANGE EVEN IF YOU DON'T KNOW THE SECRET REASONS BEHIND YOUR BEHAVIOR

A little over nine years ago one of the authors (Howard Rosenthal) received a book catalog in the mail. That in itself certainly wasn't unusual. As a professional counselor, he had received literally hundreds of similar catalogs.

Somehow this one was different. He had a really good feeling about this catalog. Why? Well it was nothing he actually could describe, just intuition. He stuck it in his top dresser drawer with this uncanny hunch that he could someday write a book for the publisher who sent out the catalog.

Sounds a bit unscientific, perhaps even a little silly. Anyway, a few years later he pulled out his catalog, which had accumulated more than its share of dust in the interim. He sent the publisher a book, which the company (Accelerated Development Inc.) decided to publish.

Now because of his ties with that company, he met an unusually creative fellow (the other author of this book) named Joseph Hollis. One day Joe had an overwhelming impulse to compose an innovative book on positive mental health. He contacted Howard who had "a good intuitive feeling about Joe's impulse." They went with the impulse and...

YOU ARE READING THAT BOOK!!!
SO...

IF YOU HAVE AN INTUITION, A HUNCH, AN INSTINCT, OR A DREAM THAT ISN'T GOING TO HURT ANYBODY ELSE...THEN GO FOR IT...JUST DO IT!

If you look closely, you'll recognize a couple of familiar faces cheering you on from the stands...

Here's to your positive mental health,

Dr. Joseph Hollis and Dr. Howard Rosenthal

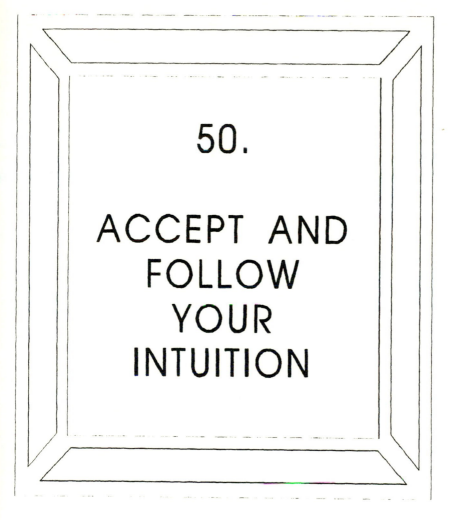

50.

ACCEPT AND FOLLOW YOUR INTUITION

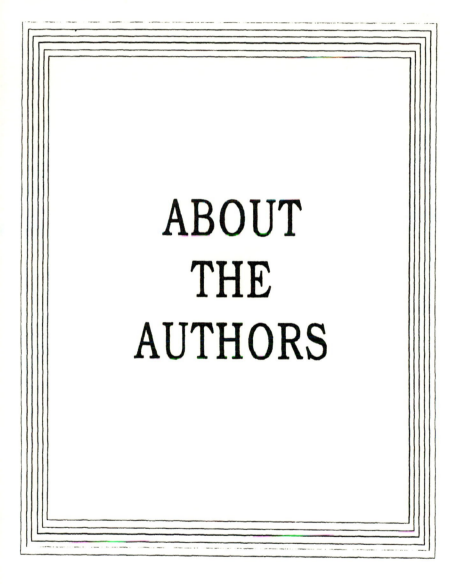

ABOUT
THE
AUTHORS

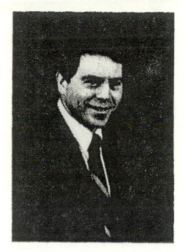

Dr. Howard Rosenthal is the author of the *Encyclopedia of Counseling* and the popular *NBCC and State Counselor Examination* audio series. Therapists nationwide use his materials to prepare for licensure and certification exams. He also wrote the innovative book, *Not with My Life I Don't: Preventing Your Suicide and That of Others* and the companion tapes, *Suicide Prevention for Young People* and *Suicide Prevention: Crash Course for Counselors and Therapists.*

He is listed in the National Directory of Distinguished Providers for Counseling and Development, Who's Who Among Human Services Professionals, Who's Who in the Midwest, and Who's Who Among America's Teachers. In 1988, he was inducted into the St. Louis Community College Hall of Fame for his accomplishments.

Dr. Rosenthal received his master's degree from the University of Missouri at St. Louis and his doctorate from St. Louis University. Over 100,000 people have heard his mental health lectures making him one of the most popular speakers in the Midwest. He has been a consultant and a guest on numerous radio and television shows. He has appeared as the expert in videos and movies and has been quoted frequently in magazine and newspaper articles.

He currently has private practices in St.Charles and St. Louis, MO., and teaches courses at St. Louis Community College and Webster University.

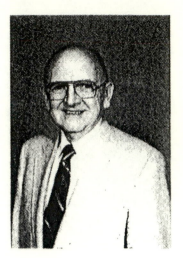

Dr. Joseph W. Hollis is Chairperson and Professor Emeritus, Department of Counseling Psychology and Guidance Services, Ball State University, Muncie, Indiana.

Certified as psychologist, private practice in Indiana, Joe is an active member in various professional activities at local, state, and national levels.

He has served as president of state guidance associations in two different states; as president of a national association (Association for Humanistic Education and Development); as Board of Directors member and senator for several years for American Personnel and Guidance Association; on the Editorial Board for the national publication, *The Vocational Guidance Quarterly*; and as a member of various committees in psychology and counseling associations.

Joe takes an active role professionally as researcher, speaker, workshop leader, and lecturer. He has special interests in individual's expectations and extent of fulfillment by different counseling techniques and theoretical positions. Career development and life planning have been a major concern to Joe, which causes him to research priorities, thrusts, and flexibility of one's energy commitments. He has researched stages of psychological regression caused by long-term unemployment.

CPSIA information can be obtained at www.ICGtesting.com
Printed in the USA
LVOW12s1146020814

397144LV00003B/128/P